NCLEX: Endocrine System

105 Nursing Practice Questions & Rationales to EASILY Crush the NCLEX!

Chase Hassen
Nurse Superhero
© 2016

Disclaimer:

Although the author and publisher have made every effort to ensure that the information in this book was correct at press time, the author and publisher do not assume and hereby disclaim any liability to any party for any loss, damage, or disruption caused by errors or omissions, whether such errors or omissions result from negligence, accident, or any other cause.

This book is not intended as a substitute for the medical advice of physicians. The reader should regularly consult a physician in matters relating to his/her health and particularly with respect to any symptoms that may require diagnosis or medical attention.

All rights reserved. No part of this publication may be reproduced, distributed, or transmitted in any form or by any means, including photocopying, recording, or other electronic or mechanical methods, without the prior written permission of the publisher, except in the case of brief quotations embodied in critical reviews and certain other noncommercial uses permitted by copyright law.

NCLEX®, NCLEX®-RN, and NCLEX®-PN are registered trademarks of the National Council of State Boards of Nursing, Inc. They hold no affiliation with this product.

© Copyright 2016 by Chase Hassen & Nurse Superhero.
All rights reserved.

TABLE OF CONTENTS

Chapter 1: NCLEX Questions, Answers, & Rationales on the Endocrine System 1

Conclusion 53

First, I want to give you this FREE gift...

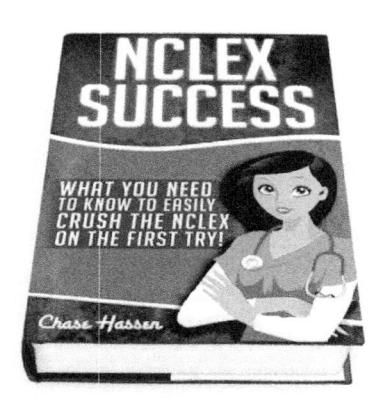

Just to say thanks for downloading my book, I wanted to give you another resource to help you absolutely crush the NCLEX Exam.

For a limited time, you can download this book for FREE.
http://bit.ly/1VvK2e7 .

CHAPTER 1:
NCLEX QUESTIONS, ANSWERS, & RATIONALES ON THE ENDOCRINE SYSTEM

When studying for the NCLEX test, it is important to take as many practice questions as possible so that you can identify areas you know well and differentiate them from areas that need more review. The following are 105 questions on the topic of the Endocrine System. Take the test and compare your answers with the questions, answers, and rationales provided below. Good luck!

1. The "master gland" in the body is which gland?
   a. Pancreas
   b. Parathyroid Gland
   c. Pituitary Gland
   d. Thyroid Gland

Answer: c. The pituitary gland is also known as the "master gland" because it makes many hormones that affect all of the other glands of the body.

2. Which is not an endocrine gland?
   a. *Ovary*
   b. *Testes*
   c. *Adrenal gland*
   d. *Liver*

   Answer: d. The ovaries, pancreas, parathyroid gland, thyroid gland, testes, and adrenal glands are all considered part of the endocrine system because they release hormones in the body.

3. In endocrinology, what is meant by a "feedback mechanism"?
   a. *When a hormone level reaches adequate levels, it feeds back on another hormone, so that the hormone decreases.*
   b. *When two hormones are at a high level, one hormone must turn off another one.*
   c. *When a hormone level is low, it causes all other hormones to be low as well.*
   d. *When the pancreas secretes enough insulin, the glucose levels drop to low levels.*

   Answer: a. When a hormone reaches adequate levels, it turns off the production of another hormone, usually a hormone secreted by the pituitary gland. For example, when T4 and T3 levels are adequate, the pituitary shuts down secretion of TSH.

4. Which is not an example of a type of hormone?
   a. Amine hormone
   b. Carbohydrate hormone
   c. Peptide hormone
   d. Steroid hormone

Answer: b. Hormones can be steroid hormones, peptide hormones or amine hormones.

5. Match the part of the pituitary gland with the correct hormone secreted by it.

   Check all that apply.

   a. Anterior pituitary—TSH
   b. Anterior pituitary—FSH
   c. Anterior pituitary—TRH
   d. Posterior pituitary—ACTH
   e. Posterior pituitary—ADH

Answer: a. b. d. The posterior pituitary gland secretes ADH and oxytocin. TRH is thyrotropin releasing hormone, secreted by the hypothalamus. The anterior pituitary gland secretes many different hormones including growth hormone, ACTH, LH, FSH and TSH.

6. The pituitary gland hormone that influences carbohydrate, protein, and fat metabolism and is responsible for the growth of cells, muscles and bones is what hormone?
    a. Thyroid stimulating hormone
    b. Growth hormone
    c. Follicle stimulating hormone
    d. Adrenocorticotropic hormone

Answer: b. Growth hormone is responsible for the growth of cells, muscles and bones and helps regulate carbohydrate, protein, and fat metabolism.

7. The pituitary hormone responsible for the release of adrenal androgens and corticosteroids is what?
    a. ACTH
    b. FSH
    c. LH
    d. TSH

Answer: a. ACTH triggers the release of adrenal androgens and corticosteroids from the adrenal cortex.

8. Which pituitary gland hormone regulates water conservation?
    a. Oxytocin
    b. TSH
    c. ACTH
    d. ADH

Answer: d. Antidiuretic hormone (ADH) is secreted by the posterior pituitary gland and is responsible for the conservation of water.

9. The thyroid gland secretes all but the following hormone?
   a. Thyroxine
   b. Parathyroid hormone
   c. Calcitonin
   d. Triiodothyronine

Answer: b. The thyroid gland is responsible for the secretion of thyroxine, triiodothyronine and calcitonin.

10. A patient has an iodine deficiency. What thyroid condition are they likely to have?
    a. Hashimoto's thyroiditis
    b. Goiter
    c. Grave's disease
    d. Medullary thyroid cancer

Answer: b. Patients with iodine deficiency tend to have an enlargement of the thyroid gland known as a goiter. This is because the thyroid is trying to enlarge in order to take up as much iodine as possible.

11. The hormone in the endocrine system responsible for O2 consumption and metabolism is what?
    a. Parathyroid hormone
    b. Thyroid stimulating hormone
    c. Thyroxine
    d. Thyrotropin releasing hormone

Answer: c. Thyroxine and triiodothyronine are both responsible for oxygen consumption and the regulation of metabolism.

12. The pituitary gland is triggered to release TSH. What affect does this have on the endocrine system?
    a. *It causes T4 and T3 to be made and released by the thyroid gland.*
    b. *It facilitates the synthesis of T3 from T4.*
    c. *It facilitates the syntheses of T4 from T3.*
    d. *It facilitates the release of calcitonin from the thyroid gland.*

Answer: a. The release of TSH causes the thyroid gland to make and release T4 and T3 in the presence of sufficient iodine.

13. The patient has an elevated calcium level. What hormone can you expect also to be high?
    a. *Parathyroid hormone*
    b. *Growth hormone*
    c. *Calcitonin*
    d. *Thyroxine*

Answer: c. Calcitonin is released by the thyroid gland in response to elevated Calcium levels. This results in an increased deposition of Calcium into the bones.

14. Parathyroid hormone results in what chemical changes in the body?
    a. An increase in phosphate and a decrease in calcium
    b. An increase in calcium and a decrease in phosphorus
    c. A decrease in calcium and a decrease in phosphate
    d. An increase in calcium and an increase in phosphate

Answer: b. The release of parathyroid hormone by the parathyroid glands causes an increase in serum calcium and a decrease in serum phosphate. Calcium and phosphate always have an inverse relationship with one another.

15. A patient has an epinephrine-secreting pheochromocytoma. What part of the endocrine system is involved?
    a. Parathyroid gland
    b. Adrenal cortex
    c. Adrenal medulla
    d. Pituitary gland

Answer: c. The pheochromocytoma is usually located in and around the adrenal medulla.

16. The patient is experiencing tachycardia, increased blood pressure, and anxiety. What endocrine hormone is likely responsible for the symptoms?
    a. Cortisol and ADH
    b. ADH and Triiodothyronine
    c. Thyroxine
    d. Epinephrine and Norepinephrine

Answer: d. Epinephrine and Norepinephrine are released by the adrenal medulla and gives tachycardia, increased heart rate and anxiety as part of the "fight or flight" response.

17. The patient has a low mineralocorticoid level. What endocrine organ is likely causing the problem?
    a. Adrenal cortex
    b. Parathyroid gland
    c. Adrenal medulla
    d. Thyroid gland

Answer: a. The adrenal cortex secretes aldosterone, which is a mineralocorticoid.

18. The patient is having a dysfunction of the adrenal cortex. Which hormones are likely to be affected? List all that apply.
    a. Epinephrine
    b. Aldosterone
    c. Cortisol
    d. Androgenic hormones
    e. Norepinephrine

Answer: b. c. d. The adrenal cortex secretes aldosterone, cortisol and androgenic hormones. Epinephrine and norepinephrine are secreted by the adrenal medulla.

19. Actions of aldosterone include any of these. Select all that apply.
    a. Sodium excretion
    b. Sodium retention
    c. Potassium retention
    d. Water retention
    e. Potassium excretion

Answer: b. d. e. The secretion of aldosterone results in sodium retention, potassium excretion, and water retention.

20. A patient has been diagnosed with Cushing's syndrome. What hormone is expected to be elevated and what does this hormone do?
    a. *Parathyroid hormone—increases the levels of Calcium in the body*
    b. *Cortisol—converts amino acids and fats into glycogen*
    c. *Epinephrine—increases heart rate and cardiac output*
    d. *Norepinephrine—increases blood pressure*

Answer: b. In Cushing's syndrome, there is an elevated blood level of cortisol, which is responsible for the conversion of amino acids and fats into glycogen.

21. People with type 1 diabetes have to take insulin because of what reasons? Select all that apply.
    a. *The pancreatic islet cells of Langerhans do not produce enough insulin.*
    b. *They have an autoimmune disease.*
    c. *They have insulin resistance.*
    d. *Cortisol is producing too much glycogen.*
    e. *They have lost the exocrine function of the pancreas.*

Answer: a. b. People with type 1 diabetes have an autoimmune disease that causes destruction of the islet cells of Langerhans in the pancreas so no insulin is produced.

NCLEX: Endocrine System

22. The hormone responsible for the metabolism of fats, proteins, and carbohydrates in the body and promotes the active transport of glucose into fat cells and muscle cells is what?
   a. Glucagon
   b. Pancrease
   c. Insulin
   d. Thyroxine

Answer: c. Insulin is responsible for the metabolism of fats, proteins and carbohydrates in the body, and promotes the active transport of glucose into fat and muscle cells.

23. Functions of insulin include the following. Select all that apply.
   a. Promote the conversion of glycogen to glucose.
   b. Stimulates active transport of glucose into fat and muscle cells.
   c. Stimulates the breakdown of fat into glycogen.
   d. Stimulates the synthesis of glucose into glycogen.
   e. Promotes the conversion of fatty acids into fat.

Answer: b. d. e. Insulin stimulates the active transport of glucose into fat and muscle cells, stimulates the synthesis of glucose into glycogen, and promotes the conversion of fatty acids into fat. It is glucagon that promotes the conversion of glycogen into glucose.

24. What is the main regulatory factor in the release of insulin from the pancreas?
    a. *Glucagon levels drop.*
    b. *Blood glucose rises.*
    c. *Glycogen levels get too low.*
    d. *Blood sugar drops.*

Answer: b. When the blood sugar rises, insulin is triggered to release from the pancreas.

25. Carbohydrates are the preferred fuel source for the body's cells. What things must be in place for this to happen? Select all that apply.
    a. *Reserve stores of glycogen are present.*
    b. *There is enough fat in the body.*
    c. *The lean muscle mass is adequate.*
    d. *Carbohydrate intake is adequate.*
    e. *There is enough insulin to put glucose into the cells.*

Answer: a. d. e. Carbohydrate can be used as the preferred source of energy if there is enough glycogen in the liver, the carbohydrate intake is adequate, and there is enough insulin to put glucose into the cells.

26. A patient has fatigue, is cold all the time, and has constipation, weight gain, and dry skin. What endocrine problem is most likely considered?
   a. Hyperthyroidism
   b. Hypoadrenalism
   c. Cushing's disease
   d. Hypothyroidism

Answer: d. The syndrome of fatigue, cold feeling, constipation, weight gain and dry skin is most likely hypothyroidism and this should be strongly considered in the differential diagnosis.

27. The symptom of excessive thirst can occur in which endocrine diseases?
   a. Hyperaldosteronism
   b. Cushing's disease
   c. Diabetes mellitus
   d. Addison's disease
   e. Diabetes insipidus

Answer: c. e. Both diabetes mellitus and diabetes insipidus can present themselves with the symptom of excessive thirst.

28. A female patient has developed exophthalmos. What endocrine condition do you think of?
    a. Addison's disease
    b. Cushing's syndrome
    c. Hyperthyroidism
    d. Hashimoto's thyroiditis

Answer: c. Exophthalmos is a classic finding in hyperthyroidism.

29. A patient has a new finding of increased pigmentation of the skin in the absence of sun or tanning bed exposure. What endocrine condition do you think of?
    a. Addison's disease
    b. Cushing's syndrome
    c. Grave's disease
    d. Hashimoto's thyroiditis

Answer: a. Hyperpigmentation is a classic finding in Addison's disease.

30. An adult patient has developed enlarged physical features including big hands, coarse facial features, and bigger feet. What hormone is likely involved?
    a. ADH
    b. Insulin
    c. GH
    d. ACTH

Answer: c. Growth hormone excesses in adults can lead to features consistent with acromegaly.

31. A patient begins to have a rapid heart rate, high blood pressure, and anxiety. What condition do you suspect might be the problem?
   a. *Hyperthyroidism*
   b. *Pheochromocytoma*
   c. *Addison's disease*
   d. *Cushing's disease*

Answer: b. A pheochromocytoma is a tumor of the adrenal medulla which can secrete epinephrine and norepinephrine, causing symptoms of rapid heart rate, high blood pressure, and anxiety.

32. A patient has a low cortisol level. What test is done to see if the problem is from the pituitary gland or from the adrenal gland?
   a. *TSH stimulation test*
   b. *FSH stimulation test*
   c. *LH stimulation test*
   d. *ACTH stimulation test*

Answer: d. The ACTH stimulation test will detect whether or not the cortisol level dysfunction is from a pituitary source (a lack of ACTH) or from an adrenal gland source.

33. The patient is having a fluid deprivation test. What blood test will be drawn to identify the positivity or negativity of the test?
   a. Parathyroid hormone
   b. Oxytocin
   c. ADH
   d. Growth hormone

Answer: c. When a patient is deprived of water, the level of ADH from the posterior pituitary gland should rise in response. The test drawn then is an ADH level.

34. A patient is having a radioactive iodine uptake test (RAI). What do you tell the patient about this test? List all that apply.
   a. This is a test to check your pituitary gland function.
   b. You will receive a safe dose of radioactive iodine before the test.
   c. The test will scan the amount of uptake of iodine in the thyroid gland.
   d. The test will check for suppression of TSH.
   e. High uptake indicates hyperthyroidism.

Answer: b. c. e. The radioactive iodine uptake test checks for over or under thyroid function. The patient receives a safe dos of radioactive iodine tracer and the amount of uptake of radioactivity is measured the next day. A high uptake indicates hyperthyroidism and a low uptake indicates hypothyroidism.

35. A 24-hour urine test for free catecholamines checks these things in the urine. Select all that apply.
    a. Metanephrines
    b. Epinephrine
    c. Aldosterone
    d. Vanyllylmandelic acid
    e. Norepinephrine

Answer: a. b. d. e. The 24-hour urine test for free catecholamines assesses the urine for free epinephrine, norepinephrine and their metabolic products, metanephrines and vanyllylmandelic acid.

36. A patient is being evaluated for the presence of diabetes mellitus. What do you tell the patient? Select all that apply.
    a. It takes two consecutive high fasting readings to diagnose diabetes mellitus.
    b. You cannot eat for 24 hours prior to the test.
    c. A fasting blood sugar of 100 mg/dL or more indicates diabetes.
    d. Eat a light breakfast before the test.
    e. A fasting reading of greater than 126 mg/dL is indicative of diabetes.

Answer: a. e. It takes two fasting blood tests of 126 mg/dL to diagnose diabetes mellitus. The patient must be fasting for at least 8 hours before the test.

37. A patient is being scheduled for an oral glucose tolerance test. You are giving the patient instructions. Select all that are accurate.
    a. The patient will be drinking a sweet liquid and will have a blood glucose test after that.
    b. If the blood glucose is greater than 200 mg/dL two hours after the test, it indicates diabetes.
    c. The patient must eat a high protein diet for three days prior to the test.
    d. The patient must be fasting for 12 hours before the test.
    e. The test may take up to 5 hours to complete.

Answer: a. b. e. In an oral glucose tolerance test, the patient must eat a high carbohydrate diet for three days before the test and must be fasting with nothing but water for 10 hours before the test. A blood glucose test of greater than 200 mg/dL indicates diabetes. The test may take up to five hours to definitely confirm diabetes.

38. A patient has a greater chance of getting an infection. What endocrine disease or diseases could they be suffering from? Select all that apply.
    a. Addison's disease
    b. Cushing's disease
    c. Diabetes mellitus
    d. Diabetes insipidus
    e. Grave's disease

Answer: b. c. People with Cushing's disease and diabetes mellitus are at a greater risk for developing infections.

39. Common conditions resulting in medical conditions are a direct result of hypersecretion of the pituitary gland. What are these conditions and matching hormone elevations? Select all that apply.
   a. TSH—hypoparathyroidism
   b. ACTH—Cushing's syndrome
   c. GH—hyperaldosteronism
   d. GH—acromegaly
   e. FSH—polycystic ovarian syndrome

Answer: b. d. The two most common conditions stemming from hypersecretion of the pituitary gland are ACTH secretion, which leads to Cushing's syndrome, and GH secretion, which leads to acromegaly.

40. A patient has had a hypophysectomy through the transphenoid approach. As his nurse, what is your responsibility postoperatively? Select all that apply.
   a. Observation for clear fluid that contains protein coming from the nose.
   b. Giving ACTH.
   c. Immediately giving T4.
   d. Observe visual acuity to check for possible hematoma formation.
   e. Nasal packing to stay in place for twenty four hours.

Answer: a. d. e. After removal of the pituitary gland (hypophysectomy) by means of transphenoid approach, the patient is observed for protein-containing clear fluid coming from the nose which might indicate CSF leakage. Visual acuity is assessed to look for possible hematoma at the site of the removed pituitary gland. Nasal packing is kept in place for 24 hours. Cortisol is given immediately after surgery to prevent an Addisonian crisis, while thyroid replacement may not need to be given for several weeks.

41. What needs to be replaced after a hypophysectomy? Select all that apply.
    a. Growth Hormone
    b. Testosterone for males and Estrogen/progesterone for females.
    c. Aldosterone
    d. T4
    e. ACTH

Answer: a. b. c. d. After a hypophysectomy, aldosterone, Growth hormone, cortisol, testosterone for males and estrogen/progesterone for females, and T4 need to be replaced. ACTH is not replaced because cortisol is already being given.

42. A patient has just been diagnosed with diabetes insipidus. What can you tell the patient in the way of patient education? Select all that apply.
    a. It is a disorder of the adrenal glands.
    b. It involves an absence of vasopressin from the posterior pituitary gland.
    c. It involves having an insatiable thirst.
    d. The patient will have a great deal of urine output.
    e. Fluid restriction will help the condition.

Answer: b. c. d. In diabetes insipidus, vasopressin is not released from the posterior pituitary gland. This results in an insatiable thirst and large volumes of urine output, despite fluid restriction, which can lead to extreme dehydration.

NCLEX: Endocrine System

43. A patient has just been diagnosed with SIADH (syndrome of inappropriate secretion of ADH). What can you tell the patient in terms of education? Select all that apply.
   a. It is a problem with the posterior pituitary gland.
   b. The patient will put out a great deal of urine.
   c. The urine will be very concentrated.
   d. The patient is at risk for hyponatremia.
   e. The patient will have an abrupt weight gain.

Answer: a. c. d. e. In SIADH, the patient will put out very little, concentrated urine and is at risk for hyponatremia. They will have an abrupt weight gain without edema and can have neurological findings, including muscular twitching, seizures, and headaches.

44. Your patient has been diagnosed with Grave's disease. What can you tell her in the way of education? Check all that apply.
   a. The thyroid gland is underactive.
   b. The thyroid gland is being attacked by immunoglobulins.
   c. You may feel jittery, nervous or tense.
   d. You run the risk of hypertrophy of the heart and heart failure.
   e. Your heart rate will be low.

Answer: b. c. d. In Grave's disease, the thyroid gland is overactive because the thyroid is being stimulated by immunoglobulins. As a result, you may feel tense, nervous or jittery and run the risk of heart failure and death from myocardial hypertrophy.

45. The patient has an overactive thyroid gland. Which of the following is not a good long term treatment for the condition?
   a. Propranolol
   b. Propylthiouracil
   c. Methimazole
   d. A dose of radioactive iodine

Answer: a. Propranolol is used prior to thyroidectomy but is not used for long term management of hyperthyroidism. Other treatment choices include giving the patient a dose of radioactive iodine, or giving propylthiouracil or methimazole.

46. The patient is having an acute attack of thyrotoxicosis. What symptoms can you expect? Check all that apply.
   a. Hypothermia
   b. Extreme respiratory distress
   c. Tachycardia
   d. Restlessness or delirium
   e. Signs and symptoms of heart failure

Answer: b. c. d. e. A patient with an acute attack of thyrotoxicosis has hyperthermia, extreme respiratory distress, restlessness progressing to delirium, tachycardia, and signs and symptoms of heart failure. This can be life-threatening.

47. A person has been diagnosed with myxedema. What is going on?
    a. They have a severe case of Grave's disease.
    b. The parathyroid glands are not functioning.
    c. They have a severe case of hypothyroidism.
    d. They have hyperthyroidism with heart failure.

Answer: c. Myxedema is another name for severe hypothyroidism.

48. What is the best blood test to screen for hypothyroidism?
    a. T4
    b. TSH
    c. T3
    d. Thyroglobulin

Answer: b. In cases of hypothyroidism, the TSH will be elevated due to the feedback loop between the thyroid gland and the pituitary gland. An elevated TSH is a sensitive test for hypothyroidism.

49. The signs of hyperparathyroidism include the following. Select all that apply.
   a. Bone hypercalcification
   b. Elevated serum Calcium
   c. Elevated serum Phosphorus
   d. Low serum phosphorus
   e. Increased urinary levels of Calcium and Phosphorus

Answer: b. d. e. A patient with hyperparathyroidism will have hypocalcification of bone, increased serum calcium, low serum phosphorus with an increase in urinary excretion of both calcium and phosphorus.

50. A patient with hyperparathyroidism needs several nursing interventions. Select all that apply.
   a. Fall prevention measures
   b. Low phosphorus diet instructions
   c. High calcium diet instructions
   d. Encourage fluid intake
   e. Give cranberry and prune juice

Answer: a. d. e. A patient with hyperparathyroidism will need to drink extra fluids to avoid renal calculi, have fall prevention measures because of decalcification of bones and risk for osteoporosis, and be instructed in a low calcium high phosphorus diet. They can receive cranberry and prune juice to help prevent renal calculi from forming.

51. A common cause of hypoparathyroidism is what?
    a. An autoimmune disease
    b. Parathyroid gland infarction
    c. Idiopathic dysfunction of the parathyroid gland
    d. Inadvertent removal of the parathyroid glands during thyroid surgery

Answer: d. The parathyroid glands, imbedded in the thyroid gland can be inadvertently lost during a thyroidectomy.

52. Nursing interventions for a patient with hypoparathyroidism include what? Select all that apply.
    a. Place calcium gluconate at bedside
    b. Check Trousseau's sign for tetany
    c. Check Chvostek's sign for tetany
    d. Give large doses of vitamin D
    e. Withhold aluminum hydroxide

Answer: a. b. c. d. Nursing interventions for a patient with hypoparathyroidism include placing calcium gluconate at the bedside, checking Trousseau's sign and Chvostek's sign for evidence of tetany, giving large doses of vitamin D to aid in calcium absorption and giving aluminum hydroxide after meals.

53. A female patient is noted to have a buffalo hump, a "moon face", purple stretch marks on legs, axillae and breasts, truncal obesity, hyperglycemia and hypertension. What possible endocrine disease could she have?
    a. Addison's disease
    b. Cushing's disease
    c. Hashimoto's thyroiditis
    d. Grave's disease

Answer: b. The symptoms of buffalo hump, a moon face, purple stretch marks, truncal obesity, hyperglycemia, and hypertension are most consistent with Cushing's disease.

54. A patient has just had a bilateral adrenalectomy for Cushing's disease. What would you be most concerned about?
    a. Hyperaldosteronism
    b. Fight or flight response
    c. Addisonian crisis
    d. Low GH levels

Answer: c. After a bilateral adrenalectomy, a patient is at risk for an Addisonian crisis postoperatively.

55. A patient has developed a tumor which causes elevated sodium levels, low potassium levels, and alkalosis. What condition does the patient likely have?
a. Hypopituitarism
b. Parathyroid tumor
c. Adrenal medulla tumor
d. Primary aldosteronism

Answer: d. If a patient develops a tumor on the adrenal cortex, he or she could be suffering from an aldosterone-secreting tumor, called primary aldosteronism.

56. A patient has hyperpigmentation, weakness, nausea, vomiting, abdominal pain, hypotension and hypoglycemia. The patient should be tested for what endocrine condition?
a. Panhypopituitarism
b. Primary aldosteronism
c. Addison's disease
d. Grave's disease

Answer: c. The syndrome of hyperpigmentation, weakness, nausea, vomiting, abdominal pain, hypotension and hypoglycemia is likely suffering from Addison's disease.

57. What things can cause Addison's disease? Select all that apply.
   a. Adrenal cortical atrophy
   b. Mineralocorticoid excess
   c. Hyperaldosteronism
   d. Autoimmune disease
   e. Adrenalectomy

Answer: a. d. e. Addison's disease can be caused by an adrenalectomy, an autoimmune disease or generalized adrenal cortical atrophy.

58. Your patient has developed adrenal cortical atrophy. What do you tell him in terms of education? Check all that apply.
   a. The condition reverses itself after several months.
   b. The patient should take in extra salt when experiencing stress, hot weather or illness.
   c. The patient and family will have to be trained in the use of emergency Solu-Cortef.
   d. The patient will be in need of lifelong replacement of hormones.
   e. Symptoms of weight gain and edema mean that the replacement of hormones needs to be decreased.

Answer: b. c. d. e. The patient will need lifetime replacement of aldosterone and cortisol. They will need to take in extra sodium when under stress, extreme heat or illness and will need replacement of hormones for the rest of their lives. If they develop symptoms of weight gain and edema, the cortisol dose is probably too high. For Addisonian crises, the patient and family will need to learn how to use Solu-Cortef for cortisol replacement.

59. Symptoms of an Addisonian crisis include which of the following? Select all that apply.
    a. Hypertension
    b. Coma
    c. Severe hypotension
    d. Vascular collapse
    e. Acute bradycardia

Answer: b. c. d. In an untreated Addisonian crisis, the patient will develop severe hypotension, vascular collapse, coma, and death.

60. The doctor has determined that the patient is having an Addisonian crisis. As a nurse, what can you be expected to do? Select all that apply.
    a. Give IV nitroprusside.
    b. Give IV normal saline with 5% dextrose.
    c. Give IV Solu-Cortef
    d. Give IV fludrocortisone — *mineralocorticoid*
    e. Give IV insulin

Answer: b. c. d. In an Addisonian crisis, the treatment is restoration of volume with dextrose, giving cortisol in the form of Solu-Cortef, and giving fludrocortisone, which is a mineralocorticoid.

61. The most common cause of a pheochromocytoma is what?
    a. *Benign adrenal medullary tumor*
    b. *Benign adrenal cortical tumor*
    c. *Autoimmune disease*
    d. *Adrenal cortical atrophy*

Answer: a. The most common cause of a pheochromocytoma is a benign adrenal medullary tumor.

62. A patient is suffering from postural hypertension, tachycardia, diaphoresis, anxiety, flushing and headache. What endocrine condition do you consider?
    a. *Hypothyroidism*
    b. *Pheochromocytoma*
    c. *Pituitary adenoma*
    d. *Prolactinoma*

Answer: b. A patient suffering from postural hypertension, tachycardia, diaphoresis, headache, anxiety and flushing should be considered as possibly having a pheochromocytoma.

63. A patient is having an acute episode from having a pheochromocytoma. As a nurse, what will you be expected to do?
    a. Give a calcium channel blocker
    b. Give IV glucose
    c. Give an alpha adrenergic blocker
    d. Give an antispasmodic

Answer: c. The preferred treatment of an acute attack involving a pheochromocytoma is to give an alpha adrenergic blocker.

64. The most common postoperative complication of surgical removal of a pheochromocytoma is what?
    a. Hypoglycemia
    b. Hypotension
    c. Hyperglycemia
    d. Fluid retention

Answer: b. The most common complication upon surgical removal of a pheochromocytoma is hypotension, which usually lasts 24-48 hours after surgery.

65. You are instructing a patient as to the use of insulin. What complications of insulin therapy do you tell them about? Check all that apply.
   a. Hypoglycemia
   b. Insulin allergy
   c. Lipodystrophy
   d. Hypotension
   e. Tachycardia

Answer: a. b. c. Complications of insulin use include hypoglycemia, insulin allergy and lipodystrophy.

66. A patient has a new diagnosis of diabetes mellitus. In explaining long term implications of having the disease untreated, you tell the patient about what? Select all that apply.
   a. Liver failure
   b. Renal failure
   c. Peripheral vascular disease
   d. Hypothyroidism
   e. Neuropathy

Answer: b. c. e. You tell the patient about the chances of renal failure, peripheral vascular disease, peripheral neuropathy, diabetic retinopathy and heart disease that can occur in the setting of untreated diabetes.

67. A hospitalized diabetic patient is found in a coma. After determining that the patient has low blood sugar, what do you do? Check all that apply.
   a. Administer glucagon
   b. Administer pressor agents
   c. Administer normal saline
   d. Administer epinephrine
   e. Administer 50% dextrose

Answer: a. d. e. In a patient suffering from insulin shock/extreme hypoglycemia, you can give glucagon, epinephrine or 50% glucose solution.

68. Which is not a finding in diabetic ketoacidosis?
   a. Dehydration
   b. Lactic acidosis
   c. Incomplete lipid metabolism
   d. Increased glycogen storage

Answer: d. In diabetic ketoacidosis, there is hyperglycemia, incomplete lipid metabolism resulting in a buildup of ketones, lactic acidosis, and dehydration.

69. Precipitating factors in getting diabetic ketoacidosis include the following. Select all that apply.
    a. Too little insulin taken
    b. Surgical stress
    c. Nausea/Vomiting
    d. Dehydration
    e. Trauma

Answer: a. b. e. Precipitating factors in getting diabetic ketoacidosis include too little insulin taken, overeating, surgical stress or traumatic stress on the body. Nausea and vomiting, and dehydration are symptoms of diabetic ketoacidosis.

70. You suspect a patient is suffering from diabetic ketoacidosis. What blood and/or urine tests can confirm the diagnosis? Select all that apply.
    a. Serum glucose level
    b. Blood pH
    c. Serum potassium level
    d. Serum or urinary ketones
    e. Serum chloride level

Answer: a. b. c. d. When diabetic ketoacidosis is suspected, a serum glucose level will be elevated, the blood pH will be low, the potassium level will be low and there will be elevated serum ketone levels with a urine test positive for ketones in the urine.

71. In diabetic ketoacidosis, the primary goal of treatment is what?
    a. To shift protein metabolism to fat metabolism
    b. To shift fat metabolism to carbohydrate metabolism
    c. To increase the blood glucose
    d. To shift liver production of ketones to glycogen

Answer: b. The primary goal of the treatment of diabetic ketoacidosis is to shift fat metabolism to the utilization and carbohydrate metabolism.

72. A patient has just been diagnosed with diabetic ketoacidosis. What is the first nursing intervention you will be asked to do?
    a. Give potassium by IV
    b. Give rapid acting insulin
    c. Administration of normal saline at 500-1000 mg over 2-3 hours
    d. Give dextrose to IV solution

Answer: c. The first step in the management is to give normal saline at a rapid rate over 2-3 hours. Then 0.45% saline should be given to continue rehydrating the patient. As the patient is being volume loaded, you give potassium to correct hypokalemia, rapid acting insulin, and dextrose to prevent hypoglycemia and to give the insulin something to work on.

73. A patient has severe deficiency of the anterior pituitary gland because of a tumor in the area. What assessments are looked for? Select all that apply.
   a. Heat intolerance
   b. Elevated blood sugar
   c. Elevated urine output
   d. Bradycardia
   e. Hypoglycemia
   f. Dehydration

Answer: a. d. e. A tumor in the anterior pituitary gland results in hyposecretion of the following hormones: ACTH, TSH, LH, FSH, and prolactin. Bradycardia and cold intolerance would happen in situations of low TSH levels; hypoglycemia would be the case in pituitary hyposecretion of ACTH, while hyperglycemia would be from hypersecretion of ACTH. Polyuria and dehydration result from a posterior pituitary disorder.

NCLEX: Endocrine System

74. A patient is scheduled to have a hypophysectomy involving an anterior pituitary gland tumor through the transphenoidal approach. What should the nurse provide In terms of perioperative instructions?
    a. The patient cannot blow his or her nose nor can they sneeze following surgery.
    b. The patient should drink at least 10 glasses of fluid on the day prior to the surgery.
    c. Don't rinse out the mouth before the nasal packing is removed on the following day.
    d. Support the patient's neck when getting out of bed.

Answer: a. Due to the risk of leakage of cerebrospinal fluid, the patient should not sneeze or blow his or her nose after surgery. They are not dehydrated so can drink a normal amount of fluids preoperatively and they can rinse their mouth out with salt solution after surgery. Support of the neck is not indicated.

75. In taking a history from a patient known to have diabetes insipidus, the nurse makes the following inquiry:
    a. Has there been any temperature dysregulation, such as feeling very hot or very cold?
    b. Has there been a change in your mood?
    c. Have you noticed a change in amount and frequency of urination?
    d. Has there been a change in sexual function?

Answer: c. In diabetes insipidus, there is a vast increase in thirst along with an increase in frequency and amount of urination.

76. The patient is being discharged from the hospital with a diagnosis of diabetes insipidus. What will you tell the patient upon discharge?
    a. Appointments for follow up are not necessary.
    b. The medication will be needed for the patient's entire life.
    c. Take fluids cautiously when under a major stressor.
    d. Diet and exercise changes might require medication changes.

Answer: b. The problem is a deficiency in ADH so that vasopressin must be taken for the duration of the patient's life. Follow up appointments are necessary and diet/exercise does not change the dose of vasopressin. Under stress, an increase in fluid intake is required.

77. The nurse is taking care of a patient with Grave's disease. What client assessments should be reported?
    a. Lethargy
    b. Exophthalmos
    c. Heat intolerance
    d. Weight loss
    e. Cold, clammy skin
    f. Bradycardia

Answer: b. c. d. A patient with Grave's disease is likely to experience exophthalmos, heat intolerance and weight loss. Lethargy, cold, clammy skin and bradycardia are not signs of Grave's disease but are signs of a low thyroid condition.

78. A patient is scheduled for a radioactive iodine uptake test. When should the nurse speak to the doctor when she hears the following comment from the patient?
    a. "I take an over-the-counter cough syrup every day."
    b. "I am a vegetarian."
    c. "I like a glass of wine with my meal."
    d. "I take a baby aspirin every night."

Answer: a. The nurse is looking for evidence that the patient is taking an iodine source. Patients taking over-the-counter cough medicines may be taking in iodide. The other sources are not iodine-containing.

79. A patient is being treated for hyperthyroidism with radioactive iodine. What should the nurse instruct the patient?
    a. One does of radioactive iodine is all that is necessary.
    b. Bodily excretions are radioactive for up to a week.
    c. Report to the doctor if you have a temperature increase or an increase in pulse rate.
    d. Symptoms of hyperthyroidism will go away after 1-2 weeks.

Answer: c. After radioactive iodine, the patient may be undertreated so they should report any increases in temperature or pulse rate. More than one dose may be required. The patient may need to have a second dose; symptoms tend to subside over a period of 3-4 weeks.

80. You are developing a care plan for a patient who has just had a thyroidectomy. What should be included in the plan?
   a. The patient should attempt to correct fluid and electrolyte imbalances.
   b. Medications should be taken to decrease the vascular supply to the thyroid gland.
   c. The patient should learn range of motion exercises for the neck.
   d. The patient should undergo measures to prevent respiratory obstruction.

Answer: d. Immediately after surgery, edema can put the patient at risk for respiratory obstructions. There are no fluid and electrolyte concerns and range of motion of the neck exercises are not attempted for several days after surgery. Medications to reduce the vascular supply to the thyroid gland are given before the operation.

81. A patient has just been diagnosed with hypothyroidism. What advice should you give the patient?
   a. Use lotion for dry skin.
   b. Keep the room temperature cool.
   c. Schedule times for rest.
   d. Take medication as needed for diarrhea.

Answer: a. The skin of hypothyroid patients tends to be very dry and needs lotion. The patient already feels cold and suffers from constipation and not diarrhea. The patient is usually lethargic and should be encouraged to get up and participate in activities.

82. The patient is suffering from myxedema. What signs indicate deterioration of the patient?
    a. A pulse and respiratory rate increase.
    b. Cold skin and chills.
    c. Difficulty arousing the patient.
    d. A patient complaint of palpitations.

Answer: c. The patient may be going into a myxedema coma, which can result in death. An increase in pulse, respiratory rate and palpitations is indicative of hyperthyroidism and it is natural for the myxedema patient to have cold skin and chills.

83. A patient with hyperparathyroidism is scheduled for a removal of a part of the parathyroid gland. What do you tell the patient?
    a. Drink at least 3000 ml of fluid each day before the procedure.
    b. Take a vitamin D supplement every day.
    c. Stay in bed as much as you can.
    d. Eat a high calcium diet.

Answer: a. These patients are at risk for calcium-containing renal calculi so they should push fluids. The calcium level is already high so a high calcium diet and vitamin D are not indicated. Bedrest is not indicated.

84. The nurse is supposed to check for Chvostek's sign to see if the patient is approaching tetany after removal of the parathyroid gland. How does she do this?
    a. Block the blood flow to the wrist.
    b. Measure the rate and depth of respirations.
    c. Listen for abnormal inspiratory breath sounds.
    d. Tap the face over the facial nerve.

Answer: d. When tapping the face over the facial nerve, a positive Chvostek's sign involves twitching of the side of the face. Blocking the flow of blood to the wrist is called Trousseau's sign.

85. A patient with hypoparathyroidism needs a diet high in calcium and low in phosphorus. What food should be recommended?
    a. Milk
    b. Leafy green vegetables
    c. Cauliflower
    d. Cheese

Answer: b. Leafy green vegetables (except spinach) have a higher calcium content and a lower phosphorus content, while milk and cheese are high in both calcium and phosphorus.

86. The nurse is evaluating a patient who has Cushing's syndrome. What should be looked for?
   a. Ineffective patterns of breathing from respiratory depression
   b. Infection risk because of altered inflammatory response
   c. Pain from nerve and tissue injury
   d. Instructing the patient as to the need for lifelong replacement medication.

Answer: b. Infections can be hard to detect because of an altered inflammatory response. Breathing and pain are normal in Cushing's syndrome and there is overproduction of cortisol, not needing replacement therapy.

87. An abnormal lab result signifying primary aldosteronism is what?
   a. A serum potassium of 3 mEq/l
   b. A serum phosphorus of 3 mg/dL
   c. A serum sodium of 130 mEq/L
   d. A serum Calcium of 12 mg/dL

Answer: a. In primary aldosteronism there is severe potassium loss with an normal or elevated sodium level. Phosphorus and calcium are unaffected.

88. You are treating a patient who has Addison's disease. What do you include in the nursing care plan?
   a. Giving diuretic medications
   b. Providing dietary instructions for a low protein, low carbohydrate diet.
   c. Monitor labs for sodium and potassium imbalances.
   d. Encourage the patient in his or her self-care.

Answer: d. These patients are missing critical mineralocorticoid and corticosteroid secretions. They suffer from low sodium and elevated potassium levels. Besides replacing their mineralocorticoids and corticosteroids, they should be regularly monitored for levels of sodium and potassium.

89. A patient is being admitted because of a pheochromocytoma. What questions do you ask pertaining to their disease?
   a. "Do you ever feel palpitations or an increase in heart rate?"
   b. "Do you have bouts of feeling extremely warm and/or flushed?"
   c. "Do you feel better when you take in simple sugars?"
   d. "Do you ever have attacks where you feel very sleepy and need to rest?"

Answer: a. In a pheochromocytoma, there are episodes of increased heart rate and palpitations due to an increase in secretion of epinephrine from the tumor.

90. A patient with type 1 diabetes is being admitted. What is a likely statement the patient might make?
   a. "I was diagnosed during my pregnancy."
   b. "I suffered from an acute attack of syncope with nausea, vomiting and abdominal pain."
   c. "I was diagnosed at age 41, when I began gaining weight and urinating more often."
   d. "I was diagnosed with a fasting blood sugar of 115."

Answer: b. Type I diabetes often comes on suddenly with syncope, abdominal pain, and nausea and vomiting. If it were diagnosed in pregnancy, it would be called gestational diabetes. Type 2 diabetes comes on gradually and patients with diabetes usually have a fasting blood sugar of more than 125 mg/dL when left untreated.

91. A patient with type 1 diabetes is having a hypoglycemic reaction. What do you notice? Select all that apply.
   a. Tremors
   b. Nervousness
   c. Marked thirst
   d. Flushing of the skin
   e. Profound perspiration
   f. Constricted pupils

Answer: a. b. e. The patient with hypoglycemia will experience tremors, anxiousness and sweating. Flushing of the skin and thirst are signs of hyperglycemia rather than hypoglycemia.

92. What would you advise a diabetic patient with regard to patient education?
    a. Keep the amount of saturated fat in the diet to less than 20 percent of total calories.
    b. Keep the body weight at about 10-15 pounds above his or her ideal body weight.
    c. Don't eat any snacks between meals.
    d. Include all macronutrients in the diet.

Answer: d. A diabetic should include carbohydrates, protein and fat in the diet with only ten percent of saturated fats allowable on a daily basis. The body weight should be as close to the ideal weight as possible. Eating several small meals during the day actually help prevent sugar spikes.

93. A patient is at risk for diabetic ketoacidosis. What symptoms should the patient be warned about? Select all that apply.
    a. Dehydration
    b. Shallow respirations which are labored
    c. Acetone smell on the breath
    d. Tremors
    e. Having cold, clammy skin
    f. Having abdominal pain

Answer: a. c. f. A patient with diabetic ketoacidosis is at risk for dehydration and abdominal pain. They have an acetone-scented breath. The respirations are not labored and they do not have tremors or cold skin.

94. Good ways of preventing hypoglycemia in a diabetic patient include which of the following?
    a. Eat a snack or meal every 4-5 hours during the day.
    b. Teach a family member as to how to inject insulin when symptoms occur.
    c. Increase insulin if you are doing moderate exercise.
    d. If symptoms occur, eat some complex carbohydrates.

Answer: a. Diabetics should make sure they eat something every 4-5 hours during the day. If a hypoglycemic reaction is suspected or confirmed, glucagon and not insulin is given and the individual should consume simple carbohydrates and not complex carbohydrates.

95. A patient wants to know about preventing complications of diabetes. What is a good piece of advice to give?
    a. Know the signs of hypoglycemia and hyperglycemia by learning how to inject insulin.
    b. Follow a prescribed diabetic diet.
    c. Keep blood glucose levels near normal levels.
    d. Talk to your doctor immediately if you have any vascular, kidney or neurological changes.

Answer: c. Long term complications of diabetes include vascular, kidney and/or neurological changes. If these things are occurring, it is already too late. To prevent complications, the diabetic must keep the blood sugars at or near normal levels.

96. You are observing another nurse giving IV NPH insulin by bolus in a patient who has diabetic ketoacidosis. What intervention should you do?
    a. Tell the nurse to shake the insulin bottle before drawing up the NPH insulin.
    b. Tell them to follow the IV bolus with 5-10 units of insulin by IV per hour.
    c. Observe the nurse for proper technique.
    d. Tell the nurse to stop giving the NPH insulin and only give regular insulin by IV.

Answer: d. Only clear regular insulin should be given by IV. NPH insulin is cloudy and should not be given in an IV bolus.

97. You are an RN in charge of an LPN on your unit. What is a good task to give to the LPN to do?
    a. Create a nutritional plan for a diabetic patient.
    b. Watch for EKG changes in a patient who had a pheochromocytoma recently removed.
    c. Teach a patient about his or her Addison's disease.
    d. Watch the blood pressure on a patient with primary aldosteronism.

Answer: d. Teaching and assessing patients with the above conditions involves an RN. Monitoring blood pressure in a stable patient with primary aldosteronism is an appropriate task for an LPN.

98. A diabetic patient has been given 6 units of regular insulin at 0730. When should the nurse watch for signs of hypoglycemia as a result of the insulin dose?
   a. 0930-1030
   b. 0800-0830
   c. 1200-1400
   d. 1500-1700

Answer: a. The regular insulin dose takes about 30 minutes to begin to act with a peak at about 2 hours. Signs and symptoms of hypoglycemia from giving regular insulin usually manifest themselves at about 2 hours post-injection.

99. Which priority item should be closely monitored in a patient who has a pheochromocytoma?
   a. Weight
   b. Glucose
   c. Blood pressure
   d. Temperature

Answer: c. Patients with a pheochromocytoma suffer from marked elevations in blood pressure due to norepinephrine release. This should be monitored closely by the nurse.

100. A patient is considered at risk for having primary aldosteronism if they have what findings?
   a. Untreated lung cancer
   b. A hypothalamic lesion
   c. A history of meningitis with peripheral neuropathy
   d. A hypertensive patient with hypokalemia not taking diuretic therapy

Answer: A patient with primary aldosteronism usually has high blood pressure and hypokalemia even when not taking diuretics therapy.

101. A patient with hyperthyroidism is being taken care of by the nurse. What nursing interventions are appropriate? Select all that apply.
   a. Giving lubricating eye drops.
   b. Providing regular, small, balanced meals.
   c. Recommend periods of time for rest.
   d. Turn up the thermostat so the patient is warm.
   e. Encourage visitors to stay and converse with the patient.
   f. Do daily weights.

Answer: a. b. c. f. A patient with hyperthyroidism often suffers from exophthalmos, which may cause dry eyes. Regular small meals keep the metabolism stable and the patient, who is likely to be anxious and jittery, should have scheduled times for rest. As weight loss is common in hyperthyroidism, they should be weighed daily. The room should be kept cool and visitation kept to a minimum.

102. A patient is known to have a posterior pituitary tumor. What nursing interventions should be undertaken?
   a. Weigh the patient daily.
   b. Limit fluids.
   c. Measure urine specific gravity.
   d. Encourage the patient to drink tea or coffee.
   e. Monitor the patient's intake and output.

Answer: a. c. e. The patient is likely suffering from diabetes insipidus due to a lack of secretion of ADH from the posterior pituitary. This results in copious amounts of urination and extreme thirst. The nurse should weigh the patient daily, measure the specific gravity, encourage fluids and monitor the patient's intake and output.

103. A patient with dehydration from diabetes is being given 150 cc/hr IV fluids. How much fluid will the patient receive after 8 hours?

Fill in the blank. _____ liters

Answer: 1.2 liters. Multiply 150 cc/hr by 8 hours to get 1,200 ml of fluid. Divide by 1,000 to transfer the number to liters.

104. A patient is given 10 units of NPH insulin at 0800. When should the nurse expect the blood sugar values to be affected by this intermediate-acting insulin?
   a. 0830
   b. 1000
   c. 1200
   d. 1500

Answer: b. Intermediate-acting insulin begins to take effect in 1-2 hours. Therefore the answer is 1000.

105. A patient has just had a thyroidectomy and is being discharged from the hospital. Which of the following instructions should be given to the patient? Select all that apply.
   a. Watch for signs and symptoms of low blood sugar.
   b. Take thyroid replacement medication as prescribed.
   c. Report to the doctor any changes such as weight changes, experiencing hot or cold, lethargy, elevated or low pulse, and dry skin.
   d. Do not take any over-the-counter medications.
   e. Have injectable dexamethasone available at all times.

Answer: b. c. The patient should take thyroid replacement medication as prescribed and report symptoms related to high or low thyroid function. Over-the-counter medications can be taken and there is no anticipation for low blood sugar or the need for dexamethasone.

CONCLUSION

I hope you received a ton of value from this book. Remember, practice makes perfect so you may have to repeat these questions.

If you enjoyed this book, would you be kind enough to leave a review on Amazon? Your reviews can help others to see what kinds of helpful resources are out there!

I'll talk to you soon and see you in the next book!

Thank you and good luck on your medical endeavors!

- Chase Hassen

Nurse Superhero

Made in the USA
Monee, IL
05 June 2022